How to Tone Up Legs & Stomach with Booty Builder Exercises for Women

Specifically Designed & Formulated for Women

Created by

Matt Lord

Table of Contents

Description

Looking for a magical women's flat stomach, lean legs, and booty builder workout in two-three weeks? Unfortunately, it does not exist. You can definitely start well in three weeks towards your goals but slimming your waistline will unfortunately take much longer. There is a famous saying among fitness experts: "The best workout is the one you're currently not doing." You frequently need to push the body in different ways to produce the best results. Thus, while classical movements such as push up and squat are the basis of any successful training program, you need to learn a lot to build up the perfect body shape and fitness level.

Some of the biggest mistakes women frequently make is to try and work out so hard at the beginning which can lead to soreness and injury and it either puts them off training or they injure themselves. The best strategy you must adopt is to slow down and learn step by step what you need to know before progressing onto more advanced training techniques.

You can start by creating a strong base, which means focusing on your hip region and cardio training, including the abdomen and back. Both muscle groups combine to shape the strength of the woman's body, and any conditioning exercise for women will be directed at both. So how can women do this all in a short period without putting too much stress on the body? To answer this and many other questions, this eBook has been designed.

The main aim of this eBook is to encourage women how she can add a routine work out for her legs, stomach, and booty to achieve the long-term results. Although it did not mean you will lose all of your fat in 2-3 weeks, the main aim is to make your body comfortable with a training routine, so being a female trainer, you can enjoy a long-lasting result on your body.

To achieve the aim the eBook focuses on,

- How to Get Lean Legs
- Understand your body type
- Tips to get the lean legs
- Tricks to get the lean legs
- Lean Legs Plan for women
- Low to moderate cardio workout?
- Exercises to get the Tone & Lean Legs
- How to Achieve a Toned Stomach and Abs
- 10 Tips to get rid of Stubborn Belly Fat
- Exercise to tone belly fat
- Booty Builder Work out plan
- Why booty training is important
- Points to consider for booty building
- Booty Muscle
- Booty builder work out plan how to build and track
- Booty builder and Nutrition
- Booty Builder Work out Exercises
- Seven days Booty builder plan

Introduction

In a society where exercise is more and more common, women become more conscious of their bodies and their health. There are so many concerns,

- Selfies
- Eating habits
- How much is the carb intake?
- Why do I not look like her?
- How can I make my legs lean?
- How can I build up my booty?

Yet these things decide how women are becoming more concerned about their personality and fitness. The critical element we need to learn here is the body structure building and fitness level are both different approaches. The concept of wellness is becoming increasingly new, especially as we are all restricted to far smaller areas than we used to.

So, if you're looking for a training program as a woman that is successful at all levels and allows you to get from top to bottom, you can take the help from this eBook. Most of the exercises explained in this eBook are very simple and easy, which you can easily add to your routine life. It is important to remember that improved fitness does not automatically mean weight loss. But if to become leaner and improving the makeup of your body are also a goal, you must burn more calories than you consume. Many of the exercises explained in this eBook should burn a lot of calories and help strengthen your muscles. Note that gradual and steady weight loss is the best way to sustain loss over time.

It is also essential to avoid an extreme diet while you are on any training program. You should also take care if you want to cut down a whole food category, such as carbohydrates or go extremely low in calories. If weight loss is also a goal, dietary adjustments in conjunction with strength and aerobic exercise can help you to lose fat, build muscle, and boost health overall.

Approach your goals in a holistic manner – so rather than only concentrating on one 'magical' task, think about everything involved in reaching an aim and bear in mind that you will need to change habits, if not lifestyle if once accomplished.

There are several different patterns in physical training, but for women and, in general, all exercises are based on the four types mentioned.

- **Aerobic Exercise**

Aerobic exercise accelerates the heart rhythm and breathing. It is an activity designed to provide cardiovascular conditioning, and it is necessary to make the body function optimally.

Burning body fat, reduced blood pressure and blood sugar levels, as well as the release of endorphins, have long been correlated with Aerobic

- **Strength Training**

Creating strength and muscle mass has a lot of advantages. Creating your muscles can make you stronger, promote bone growth, enhance balance and posture, and reduce your body's risk of stress or injury. Strength training is primarily anaerobic. Anaerobic means 'without oxygen' because the cardiovascular system cannot supply enough oxygen rapidly to your muscles.

- **Flexibility Training**

Flexibility training is frequently ignored but is vital for the success of daily and athletic movements. It is usually achieved by stretching both dynamically (actively) and statically. Building strength is critical for tight muscles and injury prevention. Yoga and Pilates are perfect examples that improve versatility in fitness training.

- **Balance Training**

Another type of fitness training frequently ignored, but balance training is essential. Working on your balance will make you more secure and avoid falls. Standing on one foot and switching between the two is a common balancing technique as you put your foot into the knee in the tree pose in yoga.

Chapter 1

How to get Lean Legs

Would you like to have slim, lean legs? In skirts, shorts, and leggings, you want to feel comfortable. And you want to feel good at the beach, not mindful of your ass and thighs. Someone once said a man looks at the legs of a woman before anything else. We all want those long beautiful legs that dancers have. The thing is, without building too much muscle, you have no idea how to eat and train to get slim legs. And no matter what common culture says: women may become too bulky for themselves.

The reality is that not everyone reacts in the same way to training. Our genetics decide the muscle fibre types we have, determine our testosterone-estrogen connection, and where we store body fat. Although weight loss is one of the best approaches to get a super toned body but through exercises as well. For women, it is good to remain in shape, tonne, and strengthen the thigh muscles. Stronger thighs will mean that you will be able to leap higher and improve your stability. It is why strengthening the legs is not an easy task, but it is important to note that to tone your legs, it is essential to have good cardiovascular health. There are a lot of exercises that can be used to tone the leg muscle, and no one activity cannot target just one particular part of the body, some exercises concentrate more on leg strength and endurance than on other parts of the body.

Understand your body type to get lean legs

If you want to learn how to get lean legs, it is crucial that you understand your body type. There are three principal body styles.

- Ectomorph-this type of body is, of course, very slim (think the catwalk models). They are tall and find it hard to put on weight and muscles. They usually have slim legs already.

- Mesomorphic – this type of body is not as slim as an ectomorphic and not overweight. They usually can gain and lose weight easily and quickly add muscle.

- Endomorphic, this sort of body, is larger. They are usually short to medium in height (but not always) with shorter arms and legs. They may quickly put on muscle and fat and find it hard to lose weight.

Tips to get the lean legs

Go to an indoor cycling class

Indoor cycling is an excellent option for toning of the leg muscles, but also for the heart and weight loss. In fact, findings from the study found that sedentary, overweight women have a decrease in body weight and fat mass in 24 indoor cycling sessions.

Find stairs

When you include stairs in your workout, you maximize the use of your thigh muscles. Because each step allows you to raise your body upwards, your leg muscles are forced to work hard.

Participate in sport

Play sports. The quick participation in many games will help shape your legs from all angles. Think sports that allow you to aerobically work your legs, such as swimming golf, soccer, cycling, and volleyball.

Balance Training

Balance training tones all the smaller muscles in the legs and thighs, tightens them quickly, making them perfect, slender legs. A good strategy is to try one-legged deadlifts on the ball to really test your balance.

Strength training

Include strength training two or three days a week. It is essential to focus on a variety of exercises, including quadriceps, hamstrings, calves, and adductors, that recruit many leg muscles. Work on increasing muscle endurance and tone over muscle bulk by adding lighter weights to fatigue the legs 12 to 15 times. Start with your body weight and add weight to most exercises as you improve. Total one or two workout sets. Outstanding leg training can include calf raises, squats, lunges, lateral leg lifts, and burpees.

Interval training

While long-term exercise helps you lean your body, higher intensity exercise also allows you to burn the leg fat. Interval preparation requires a short but extreme bursts of energy coupled with minor rest periods to prepare you for the next burst of energy. High-intensity exercises are performed once or twice a week for 30 to 45 minutes. Sprint for a minute followed by two minutes of jogging or walking. Repeat 8-10 times and have a warm-up and a cool-down. The less fat your body has, the slimmer your legs will look.

Cardiovascular exercise

HIIT consumes calories and strengthens your core. This also contributes to reducing body fat. Both high-intensity interval training (HIIT) and stable aerobic training are included in your overall fitness schedule. Consider adding one session of aerobic exercise to your workout schedule for more advanced training and calorie burn. The CDC recommends that adults get at least 150 minutes of aerobic activity at moderate intensity, or 75 minutes of aerobic exercise at high intensity, per week. Combine moderate and intense aerobic exercise to achieve optimal physical fitness.

Tricks to get lean legs

- If you have broad thighs and want to slim your legs, do not lift heavy weights when performing strength exercises. For as long as you lift weights with legs or do leg exercises, the muscles on your legs are impossible to lose.

- While you train with light weights and high reps, you are not going to lose your muscle, However you are not really going to develop new muscle either, but you keep the muscle you've got.

- CrossFit and HIIT are two workouts used to bulk the muscles. While these are fantastic exercises, they are not going to give you the long, slender and lean legs you want.

- Begin your morning with a walk. One right way to sneak 10 km a day is to set your alarm a bit earlier and walk as soon as you wake up. It not only gets it done early, but it is more effective to burn fat when you do morning cardio.

- Split it up. Try to walk 5 km in the morning and try to cover the other 3-5 km all day long by walking more than you usually would.

- Follow your performance. Use the free fitness apps to keep track of your steps and kilometres. You can also download several free applications on your phone to help you track your distance and achieve those goals. You will feel encouraged to continue your training by monitoring your success.

- Keep a record when you measure your legs.

- Muscle-reinforcing workouts at least two days a week will help you lose calories, reduce fat mass, and strengthen your thighs. Include lower-body movements like squats, lunges, wall chairs, inner/outer thigh lifts, and step-ups with your body weight only.
- Keeping the reps high (at least 15 reps per set) is key to strengthening the legs without bulking. Perform three exercise rounds with minimal rest in each movement.
- It is also possible to incorporate upper body movements to your lower body workouts for a perfect two-in-one exercise. For instance, take some dumbbells or household objects to use as weights and perform the lunges with a bicep curl and squats with an overhead press of the shoulders.

Chapter 2
Lean Legs Plan for women

First of all, the most important point is that exercise alone won't give you those perfectly shaped, lean, and slender legs if you eat a lot of high in saturated fat foods such as doughnuts and potato chips. To get the look you want, you must:

- Eat a balanced, whole-food diet.
- Walking/cardio every day (30 minutes).
- Stretching on all days is just as necessary as exercise.
- High-intensity workouts (HIIT) at least twice a week.
- Do strength training 2 to 3 times a week (upper body).

Few tips before starting the exercise plan

1. The best and quickest way to build lean muscle is your lower body. You have more than 200 muscles in your lower body in addition to the body's biggest muscle — the gluteus muscles. You can keep your lower body in control by controlling the glutes. There is a huge variety of exercises to work out with the glutes, such as to stand on one leg when you are doing a squat. The harder you work, the sooner you can see results.

2. Work on the weaker side first, which for most of us is the left side. The best approach always starts each exercise from your weaker side first. If, as with lunges, you always work from the weaker side, but you may unconsciously start from your stronger side in this situation, you don't give your vulnerable side the extra attention it deserves.

3. One of the best exercises for the legs is lunges, which form the legs perfectly. For lunges, you take a straddled stance position in such a way to keep one leg forward and one leg behind you and make sure your front foot is flat on the floor. Bend your front knee so your knee covers your toes but not past them, and your back leg will slightly bend towards the ground, try not to let it touch the floor. Do ten pulses (a few inches up and down) before switching to the opposite leg. Make sure you hold your chest up. One variation of the lunge position is to lift onto the balls of the feet, this should incorporate the calves as well as on the thighs and hamstrings.

How To Get Lean Legs In 3 Steps

More Efficient Exercise – Low to a moderate aerobic intensity like fasted walking is necessary to keep your legs lean.

Know Your Body Type -To get the lean legs, you must know your body type, which tells you what sort of resistance training you can select.

The Correct Diet For Your Body Type – A balanced diet can help you lose body fat and slimming of your legs.

What Exactly is a Low to Moderate Cardio Workout?

Your body produces energy in two simple ways: anaerobic (oxygen-free) and aerobic. As your body uses the anaerobic pathway, it utilizes creatine phosphate and glycogen (carbohydrates) for generating energy.

- Your body should use the anaerobic pathways for high-intensity exercise (including high-intensity cardiovascular exercise such as running), weight training, and interval exercises.
- The aerobic pathway should be used by the body: low-intensity exercise (including low-intensity cardio, like walking). Low-intensity exercise burns fat, and it is therefore highly relevant to complete to get skinny legs.

If we speak of low to moderate cardiovascular workout, I primarily talk about walking.

The best types of cardio for lean legs are:

- 35-45 minutes walking
- 35-45 minutes of cycling
- Jogging

Walking

Walking is the most reliable form of exercise to achieve slim legs. It will help you to rid your legs of excess fat and lean them out.

Walking burns an impressive number of calories. Nonetheless, it is essential to note that prolonged, slow aerobic (e.g., walking) is not the main goal to lose weight in general. The main focus here is how to achieve slimmer more toned legs. When you do cardio at a low to moderate intensity your body first burns glycogen (carbs), and then fats. The more you exercise, the more fat your body burns. By walking longer, your body can burn more fat and help you get lean legs. The longer you go, the more fat you are burning, and the faster you are getting lean, toned legs.

However, you will also accumulate cardio periods throughout the day too.

For example, you can walk for 6 x 10 minutes every day, which is 60 minutes cardio.

It is imperative to ensure that you perform your cardiovascular exercise on a flat surface. Walking uphill uses the quadriceps and glutes which can induce bulkiness. Seek to stop the elliptical / cross-trainer and incline to the treadmill. There are many women who try this, although this strategy burns more calories than walking on a flat surface, you build muscle, and it is not going to help you get those lean legs. Better workouts can be done to develop muscles and support the whole body and better cardiovascular work can be done to strengthen your legs.

Walking vs. Running

Running consumes plenty of calories, and the net weight loss is perfect. Running, however, does not seem as right as walking for thinner legs. If it is your intention to slim down your thighs, you will need to concentrate mostly on walking and add a little running.

Eat Well

You must eat well to reduce your overall body fat if you want to get slimmer legs and get rid of the excess fat from the legs, you must eliminate bad calories from your everyday diet. You can walk a lot and do all the right workouts, but if you do not have a balanced diet and don't consume the right amount of food, then you won't get results.

To lose weight and slim your legs, you will eat less than your body requires. Below are some tips to keep the diet healthy:

Count Calories For One Week – How many calories we consume is usually not taken into account. In just one week, you need to count calories to get an idea of how much you consume. If you determine how many calories you need to consume to lose weight, this will be the best approach.

Don't Be Too Restrictive –There is no need to count long-term calories. Keep it up to a week so that you learn more about what you eat so that it can lead to a healthier food relationship.

What to eat

- Eat as much fresh and unprocessed food as possible. Try to consume plenty of fresh fruits and vegetables.
- Do not overeat, have three main meals a day and healthy snacks to keep the blood sugar stable (eat every 3-4 hours).

- Cut out all deep-fried food, vegetable oil and as much milk and soy as possible.

- Stick to healthy fats, such as extra virgin olive oil, flaxseed oil, avocados, nuts etc. don't be fooled by 'low fat' foods as these can contain hidden sugars.

- Often read food labels and avoid items containing additives such as preservatives, colours, etc.

- In the mornings, boil water (1-2 litres) and drink it warm. It is a simple Ayurvedic treatment for detoxifying, reducing hunger attacks, and enhancing peristaltic movement.

Know your hormone profile.

You will find it fascinating to learn from nutritionists and endocrinologists that your hormonal profile is responsible for storing the fat of your body and that hormonal imbalance can contribute to weight gain (or losses), especially in women. The female hormones estrogen predominance / low progesterone is partially responsible for women to hold fat around the stomach, thighs, and hamstrings.

Chapter 3

Exercises to get Toned Legs

Step Up

Stand with your feet hip-width apart, one step in front of a bench or sturdy object, arms by your side. Step up onto the bench with a leading leg, lift your opposite leg and put it on the bench, you should be standing with both your feet on the bench. Step off the bench and repeat with the same leading leg until you have finished the set, then change the leg you step up with.

Step Up Knee Raise

Stand with your feet hip-width apart, one step in front of a bench or sturdy object, arms by your side. Step up onto the bench with a leading leg, lift your opposite leg but rather than putting it on bench, lift your knee into the air so it is 90 degrees to your body. Lower the floating leg back to the ground and land firmly.

Repeat until you have finished the set, then change sides.

Lateral Step-up

Stand with your feet hip-width apart next to a bench or sturdy object, arms by your side. Step up onto the bench with the foot closest to the bench, lift your opposite leg but do not put it on the bench, you should be standing with your feet parallel but with only one foot on the bench. Lower the floating leg back to the ground and land firmly.

Repeat until you have finished the set, then change sides.

Lateral Turn Jumps

Stand on one foot, arms by your sides and slightly bend your knee in a ready to jump position. Jump to your side and extend the opposite leg and land on the other foot but facing 90 degrees out. Reset your stance and continue the movement in the opposite direction, alternating sides, smoothly and evenly. Always try to land gently, bend your knees and thighs to absorb the pressure from your muscles — not your articulations.

Walking Lunges

Before carrying out a sequence of walking lunges, your lunge technique should be perfect: Stand with your legs in hip-width position and take a large step forward on the right foot. The front (right) knee will be above the ankle and not in front of it. Make sure the knee points slightly outside and press the heel and the foot down. Bend the back (left) leg so that the knee floats over the ground. Your hips should be square and your glutes and back are straight ready for the next rep. Make sure that your body weight is right behind the front heel and keep the shoulders pulled back.

Try to complete around 10 reps per leg or set an area of approximately 20 meters. Repeat three times. Take around three to five seconds to sink into the lung before you reach the next one.

You can also add a few pulses into your buttocks for another 5-10 seconds if you want to work harder.

A walking lunge operates several leg muscles simultaneously. In fact, maintaining balance and moving correctly during the exercise also stimulates the heart and stabilizer muscles. These should work the quads, buttocks, glutes, hamstrings, and calves. Any cardiovascular session should involve a lunge sequence. Climbing stairs work with the same lunge muscles. (Good news for women too, it trains the pelvic floor automatically).

Lying Leg Raise

This exercise is suitable for indoor and outside and provides you with super firm lower abs as a bonus. Lie on your back, arms by your sides, palm-facing down. Lift both legs straight from the ground to the ceiling as slowly as possible. Stop for a second and slowly lower your legs down to the table. Using ankle weights will help make this exercise more effective.

Side Leg Raise

Lie on your side, which is a straight line from your shoulders to your ankles. Keep a small support ball between your ankles and hold your legs in place. Raise both legs and the ball as high as possible and slowly go back to the starting spot. Do all reps on one side, then switch sides and repeat. Squeeze ball the ball tightly to activate the inner thighs during the raise.

Inner Thigh Leg Lift

This routine works both on the inner and outer thighs and the booty. Sit on your left booty cheek and keep up your upper body with your hands. Cross the left-right knee. The left leg is straight to stick out. Stretch your bottom foot and raise your left leg as far as you can to the ceiling. The motion in this exercise is slow, so don't worry if you can't lift your leg far. Do not let your leg hit the floor when you pass. Match the other leg with it.

Donkey Kicks

Lay on a mat on all fours. Keep your foot relax. Now, kick-upwards to the ceiling as if you are trying to put your foot's sole on the ceiling. Try to keep your thighs parallel to the floor. Squeeze the glutes and go back to begin again. Repeat for the other side.

Banded Walks

Tie a medium resistance band around your ankles and stand in a quarter squat or athletic stance with your feet a little wider than the shoulder-width apart, toes forward or slightly out of alignment. Move one foot out to the side, keep your body upright (not sluggish), knees squatted and follow with your trailing foot. Repeat for reps in the same direction, then turn around on the opposite side.

Crossover Step-up

Pick a bench or sturdy object around the height of the knee. With one foot step up onto the bench, placing the foot squarely on the bench, toes pointing forward. With the other foot, step it over the bench and place down onto the floor on the other side of the bench with a slightly wider than shoulder width stance. Once complete on one side, lift your foot and step over the bench and return to the start position, that is 1 rep. Compete for a rep range where it challenges you but are still comfortable and can complete with perfect form. Repeat for the alternate side. If possible, do this in front of a mirror to observe your form. Dumbbells can also be used to increase the difficulty of this exercise.

The Bird Dog

This exercise deals with the core muscles, quads, hamstrings, glutes, and lower back. It is always perfect for a balancing challenge. You may have to perfect your balance at first to maintain the correct form. Start on your hands and knees, hands extended over the width of the neck. Hold your head, neck, and back in a straight line. Extend your right arm forward, as if you are going to grab something. Kick the left leg behind you at the same time until it is straight and torso-like. Hold for a count of one. You should add ankle weights to this exercise once you have perfected your balance. Return to start. Keep repeating until you have finished the set, then change sides.

Chapter 4

How to Achieve a Flat Stomach and Toned Abs

Losing the fat around your mid-section can be a battle. In addition to a risk factor for many illnesses, you can still feel bloated and depressed with excess abdominal fat. Fortunately, some techniques have proven especially successful in getting rid of excess belly fat. The most important question for women is:

"How can I quickly tone my stomach?"

There are many reasons behind this question, you might think about the harmful effects of excess fat or just want to look healthier. The good news is there are efficient ways to improve the strength of muscle and get toned abs. If you dream of a flat stomach, this section could be just what you need. Our main goal is to teach you how to burn your stomach fat best and realistically so that you can finally flaunt your stomach well.

Tips to get rid of Stubborn Belly Fat

Reduce Calorie Intake

This is a well-known fact that excess calories must be cut to cause weight loss. One common approach is to reduce the daily consumption by 500–1000 calories leads to an approximate loss of 1–2 pounds a week (0.5–1 kg). The most critical point, it can be harmful to limit the consumption of calories too much. Eating too little calories can cause a substantial decrease in your metabolic rate or daily burning of your calories. In one test, a group of people who eat 1,100 calories per day has decreased their metabolic rate more than twice as much as they did four consecutive days of intake of about 1,500 calories per day. In fact, even after you start eating like you usually do, this decrease in metabolic rate can continue. It is, therefore, critical that you do not limit your calorie intake too much or too long.

Change your Diet

You probably already know that hindered starches and saturated fat turn into belly fat. Change your diet and remove these foods as soon as possible from your diet. Substitute good fats like olive oil, nuts, and avocados for them. Furthermore, eat complex carbs such as sweet potatoes, wheat bread, and brown rice.

The amount of protein you are currently eating will possibly have to be increased. For overall health, the minimum amount of protein is around 0.36 grams per pound of your total body weight. For example, if you weigh 125 pounds, that would be 45 grams of protein a day. Your protein count will need to be increased to build muscle for toned abs. If your current diet and exercise do not give you results, raise your protein intake by approximately 1 gram per pound of bodyweight or 125 grams of protein if you weigh 125 pounds. Each of your main meals, along with snacks, will concentrate on high-protein foods such as pork, lean beef, poultry, tofu, beans, egg whites, cottage cheese, yogurt, part-skim cheeses and nuts.

Eat six small meals a day

The secret to regeneration and removal of abdominal fat is a dietary improvement. Start with five or six meals a day. When you eat a big meal and have a long gap in between meals, your body will think you are hungry and store most of the calories as fat.

The best approach is to eat your day's biggest meal at breakfast within 30 minutes of waking up. During the day, it is also essential to drink plenty of water to reduce water retention, helps to digest food and leave you feeling fresh.

Eat more soluble fibre

Soluble fibres, absorb significant quantities of water and slow food movement through the digestive tract. This has proven to prolong the emptying of the stomach, allowing the stomach to expand and render you full. In addition, soluble fibres will decrease the number of calories the body can consume from food. You are also unlikely to build up fat around your organs by consuming soluble fibre, which reduces your waist circumference and your risk of various diseases. One research found that every

10-grams increase in the daily soluble fibre intake reduced by 3.7 percent over five years the fat gain in the mid section. Oats, flaxseeds, avocados, legumes, brussels sprouts and blackberries are healthy sources of soluble fibres.

Do Aerobic Exercise

Performing fitness or aerobic exercise is a smart way to balance calories and improve health overall. Studies have also shown that it works very effectively to boost the reduction of the waistline. Research usually recommends average weekly aerobic exercise of 150–300 minutes, which is around 20–40 minutes a day. Definitions of exercise include running, walking quickly, cycling, and rowing. Adding exercise to your workout routine helps you improve your diet and maximize resistance training. Aerobic exercise helps you burn more calories, which is crucial when focusing on the tone of your muscle.

Thanks to the fat burning capacity of the exercise, fat overlaying your stomach muscles will also decrease much more rapidly if you incorporate exercise to your diet and resistance training. You will improve this toning by at least doing some of your high-intensity aerobic interval workouts. These HIIT exercises mix fewer energy consumption bursts with slightly more extended periods of moderate activity. (For example, one minute sprint, two minutes gentle jog and repeat this pattern over your cardio length).

Bloating

So many women suffer from bloating and wonder how to get rid of the bloating feeling. A bloated stomach is something that makes you feel very uncomfortable. Although bloating can be caused by several different factors, it is mostly due to incorrect digestion and poor food choices. Certain factors can include consuming too much, drinking carbonated beverages or over-eating. Apple cider vinegar is an effective way to help avoid bloating by adding one tablespoon into a glass of water and take before every meal.

HIIT

A flat stomach also reduces the body fat percentage. HIIT has proven to be one of the most powerful methods for the shredding of fat. HIIT is really straightforward. You conduct fewer workouts at a short duration, each workout is performed at a higher intensity than a regular workout. Short 30-60 second bursts of maximum effort followed by 30-120 seconds of a lower intensity to recover before the next high intensity bursts of effort. By increasing your heart rate, you speed up your metabolism and increase the burning of the body's fat.

More Standing Exercises

Doing exercises while standing up will do your wellbeing better than doing the same activities while seated or using weight machines. You trigger more muscles by standing to retain balance and maintain weight. You would then spend more time working out.

A Research comparing the results of standing and sitting exercises found that some standing exercises improved the activation of muscles by 7-25% as opposed to sitting.

Another study indicated that standing would increase breathing in comparison with sitting. Although it can seem like a small improvement, it may improve your core.

Walk at least 30 minutes daily

A healthy well balance diet and exercise combination is possibly the most successful way to achieve weight loss and improve your overall health. Ironically, studies have shown that you do not have to work out actively to support your health. Normal, vigorous walks have shown to reduce the total body fat and fat around your stomach effectively. It has been linked to a significant reduction in harmful stomach fat and a slimmer waistline for 30–40 minutes (approximately 7 500 steps) per day.

Smarter workout

One hundred crunches a day does not lead to a flat stomach. Toned abs come from a variety of exercises to help the body lose fat by increasing your heart rate in various ways. To achieve a better mid-section, you need to use a more balanced approach and apply exercises other than crunches to achieve the results. You can combine power sessions (which target the heart and entire body) with HIIT (to melt fat off) to achieve these objectives.

Drink Water

There are many ways water can help you make your stomach flat. It can help with weight loss by increasing the metabolic rate temporarily. Before meals, drinking water will help you feel better, and you can eventually have fewer calories to consume. It could also help to alleviate constipation and minimize stomach bloating. Try to drink a large glass of water before every meal.

Reduce stress levels

Stress and anxiety are very normal, and most people feel them. Stress is associated with the development of many diseases, and it is also a common cause that people continue to eat or binge, sometimes without hunger. Stress also causes the body to generate a stress hormone called cortisol, which affects the appetite and contributes directly to the accumulation of bowel fat. It can be particularly harmful to women who already have a wide bum since, in reaction to stress, they generate more cortisol, which increases the gain in body fat. You can try to incorporate other stress-relieving practices such as yoga or meditation in your daily routine. Strengthening your heart rate and other abdominal exercises will improve your overall health and appearance.

Chapter 5
Exercises to Tone Stomach Fat

Running or walking

Running or walking are exercises that not only help you shed weight from the belly; it also removes weight from other regions. Running and walking are two of the best workouts for fat burning. Therefore, a decent pair of running shoes is the only equipment you need. Between the two, running consumes more calories as compared to walking. Running and walking should be part of your strength training, so do not forget to add them in if you exercise for weight loss.

Plank

You either love it, or you hate it, it is a significant exercise to tone your stomach. Planks are a build-up movement that is done for time instead of repetitions. Place your forearms shoulder width apart on the floor and raise onto your toes, separating your knees from the floor. Contract your abs and lengthen the spine by looking just beyond your hands while you hold this position. The goal is to keep your body straight from your knees to the top of your head for a certain amount of time or in good condition if you can.

Hanging Leg Raises

It is a typical workout you probably always see in the gym. Hanging leg raises are a challenge to the lower abdomen. It is achieved by raising the knees up to the chest while hanging vigorously from a bar. The goal is to try to pull the abs solely through the lower body to the chest instead of using momentum or swing. The workout can also be performed with legs extended for further movement.

Mountain Climbers

Adopt the plank position but resting on your hands rather than your forearms, with your body straight between the top of your head and your heels. Drive your right knee to your chest and then go back to your starting point. Repeat on the opposite side, then start alternating sides for 60 seconds in fast succession.

Bicycle Crunches

Burning body fat is half the fight. Next, the abdominal muscles need to be strengthened. In a recent report, exercises from best to worst were graded. Bicycle Crunches ranked # 1 because it includes abdominal flexibility, body rotation, and more abdominal muscle activity. Lay on your back with hands behind your head. Raise your knees to your chest as you lift your head and shoulder off the ground. Move the right elbow to your left knee and straighten the right leg. Move the left elbow to your right knee and straighten the left leg. Continue swapping sides.

Ball Crunch

This movement requires a lot of relaxation that needs more muscles. You are going to need a fitness ball. Lie on the ball so that your lower back is supported, and feet are firmly planted on the ground—position hands across your chest or behind the head. Contract abs and raise your body back-up and forth – Keep your body and the ball steady through each crunch –exhale as you crunch.

Cable Crunch

Cable crunching creates continuous stress throughout the entire process, which separates this crunch variation from others. Place the rope attachment or two handles on a high pulley and kneel a few feet in front of the pulley system. Hold your palms into the rope or handles facing each other, and keep your palms tight by your head as you do the workout. Exhale and lower to the floor, pulling with your abdominals instead of arms. When you crunch, try raising your elbows right above your knees. Move to the starting position gradually, keeping your hands close around your head.

Heel Touch

Lay with your feet about the hips-width and bend your knees around 45 degrees in front of your toes. Tense your core in this position and move the left hand to touch the left heel and then return to the centre. Repeat on the other hand and keep alternating sides.

Side Plank

Lay on your side resting on your elbow. The shoulder will be over the elbow directly. Lift your legs and raise your hips to build a straight and stable head-to-heel line.

Keep your neck long, your shoulders down. During the exercise, keep your abs contracted.

Heavy Compound Exercises

Heavy compound exercises are complicated exercises which require many joints and muscle movements. Squats, deadlifts, and standing overhead presses are only a few examples of compound exercises. Although these are not particular stomach exercises, performing the movement of compound exercises with heavyweights, good form, braced core, and correct breathing results in core activation and increased overall core strength. Heavy compound movements paired with core exercises are a healthy way to strengthen your abdominal muscles.

Abdominal Crunch with legs raised

Lay on your back, hip-width apart with your legs bent and feet flat on the ground. Place your hands over your chest. Pull your knees slowly into your chest and keep them bent at 90 ° until your buttocks and your tailbone lift from the floor. Perform a crunch up to your knees, hold the position for a second and gradually lower. Carry out twelve crunches.

Half get up

Lying on your back, take the kettlebell in your right hand and stretch your right arm fully above your head. Bend your left knee with foot flat on the ground. The right leg is flat on the floor. That is the starting point. Crunch up from here with your abs and lift your left forearm to your left side, palm pressed firmly to the ground. You want to keep the right arm extended with the kettlebell throughout the whole movement. Return gradually to your starting spot and repeat for repeats then switch sides.

Dead bug

The dead bug exercise helps boost both core stability and strength, resulting in a stronger stomach. Lie on your back with your legs raised and your knees bent, your arms above your head, shoulder width apart. Contract your abs and stretch out your right arm and left leg until you almost hit the floor. Stop briefly and go back to the starting spot and switch sides, repeat for reps.

Chapter 6
Booty Builder Workout Plan

I think it is fair to say most ladies like a perky, round and robust booty. Some of us are born with greater genes, while others are not so lucky. A lifted, curvy, and strong booty we all like, right? Could one be acquired without the right genetics? Totally! While genetics can go a long way to build your natural curves, the right exercises and diet will significantly improve your booty. The fact is to build the booty; it is a straightforward collection of basic exercises that you need to perform with increasing strength. Another thing you should note is that the booty, otherwise known as gluteus is just another muscle, which makes the workout easy and provides excellent results without the need for cosmetic surgery or years of preparation.

There is more to building and toning muscle than just working out. Health is a significant component of it. Notice I did not say "diet." If your goal is to firm and build muscle, you must fuel your muscles properly. Not consuming enough will not only slow down your monthly cycle but also interrupt your metabolism, which causes your body to maintain excess fat. You should, of course, always talk to a health care provider before modifying your diet, as these are just general recommendations.

Why booty training is important

Our glute muscles are relaxed during daily tasks like walking or bending to pick something up as our other muscle classes. And because we spend so much time sitting, over time, our glute muscles will actually get weaker. This booty training will help people to strengthen their glutes and hamstrings over and over again.

Points to consider for booty building

You need to consider the following points before starting the booty building work out.

- **Strength and Resistance training**

You need to practice strength and resistance training with intensity to build progressive overload. The key to ensuring that your muscles are growing is to force your body to adjust. The only way to do that effectively is to concentrate on becoming better during your workouts. In short, by continually strengthening your muscles over time, building a consistent progressive overload (including adding weight to the bar).

- **You must eat enough to develop muscle consistently**

Muscles can only grow in the presence of a caloric surplus adequately generated. I highly suggest for women that your caloric surplus does not exceed 300 calories per day. Your training experience is also significant.

- **Rest and Recovery**

Rest and recovery are very important after every training session if you want to train again, your body must repair itself. And if you are not as tired or have enough time off during the week in order to heal your body, you can always try different workout exercises.

Booty Muscle

The booty (gluteal muscles) consists of 3 muscles, out of which two are really important.

- **Gluteus Maximus**

The Gluteus Maximus stretches the hip/leg backward. Because this muscle is very large, you should primarily concentrate on overloading this muscle as you attempt to expand your booty because it will reach the maximum growth potential.

- **Gluteus Medius**

The Gluteus Medius is responsible for the abduction that raises the thigh and to flex and rotate the hip. Movements like side-lying clams can support the medium gluteus.

- **Gluteus Minimus**

The Gluteus Minimus is the smallest and least important booty muscle. It is situated immediately beneath the Gluteus Medius muscle. The Gluteus Minimus works alongside the Gluteus Medius to abduct the thigh and supporting the body on one limb.

Booty builder work out plan

There are many ways in which you can build a system that works for you. Depending on your goals, you can train twice a week, or you can train six days a week, concentrating on different body parts for each session.

It is all up to you, certain considerations need to be taken into account when choosing a suitable fitness schedule for you. There are a few factors to be considered when deciding how many days you will have to work out a week:

- Work schedule.
- The time it takes to get to the gym.
- How much time you will spend in a gym.
- What are your goals?
- How much experience you have in fitness rehabilitation capacities?
- It is normal to follow the whole body or the upper / lower split system from beginners to advanced trainees for 3 to 4 days a week.
- Proper rest is essential, as you want to make sure that you rest the same muscle group at least 48 hours between training. For example, after you train the booty program, you will wait 48 hours to train it again, but within that time frame, you can train other exercise routines. I recommend two full days of rest each week, however you can make them days a recovery day, such as yoga, swimming, etc. Nothing heavy. Nothing vigorous.

Tracking your progress

It is important and highly motivating during the work out cycle. When taking progress photos, keep in mind:

- Take pictures at the same time each week.
- Use the same clothes and the same light every week.
- Use "before" photos before beginning the plan.
- Set a reminder on your phone every four weeks to take new photos.
- Make sure that your photos are full-length body pictures.

Nutrition and booty builder workout

For muscle growth, the diet is crucial. Here are a few of the suggestions in terms of your diet:

- Make sure that you consume plenty of calories for proper muscular growth. The typical recommendation is 1 gram per pound bodyweight for protein intake. If you weighed 120 lbs, for example, the advice is 120 g of protein daily.
- Eat around the time of your workout is essential. It is usually recommended a meal of at least 50 g of carbs and 30 g of protein within one hour before your workout. The same goes for an hour after the workout; a meal is crucial to help strengthen the muscles. You can also drink a protein shake right after, but you will also need a snack.
- The best time to have a treat is after exercise; the muscles are more likely to benefit. Eat a cookie if you like a treat!
- You must have enough protein to eat! One gram of protein should be consumed per each pound of body weight as a

typical guideline per muscle development. Lean meats, bacon, Greek yogurt, and protein supplements/shakes are some healthy sources of protein.

- A significant amount of dietary fat comes from the origins of protein (salmon, eggs, nuts). Healthy fats will help you live healthier and help you lose weight while the protein forms and tones your body.

- Another critical factor is ensuring that you must eat something healthy after a workout. The bulk of muscle development happens after the exercise is done. Which means, for example, another part of a protein, but also a good dose of dense carbohydrates and nutrients. There will be a few examples: full-grain bread, brown rice, sweet potatoes, and most fruit/veggies.

Chapter 7

Booty Builder Workout Exercises

You need to speak to your doctor if you are not physically fit before taking part in a new workout regimen. I want you to be as safe as you can because you must push yourself when it comes to the actual preparation. Your number one goal will always be the right type of exercise and workout plan. Before you start, make sure you know exactly how to do the exercise. Lifting heavy weights puts the muscles under stress, so you must know how to manage yourself. The human body must be required to adjust to stress, which is above the limit so as to allow a muscle to expand, develop strength and increase efficiency.

If you want to grow your booty (or any other muscle groups), you will have to continuously overwhelm the muscle group by training with weight and gradually increasing the strength over time. Heavy weightlifting will not make you bulky. The female body can not contain enough testosterone to render you overly muscular. Nonetheless, lifting heavy weights gives your booty a natural boost and makes it tight and firmer. Sounds good?

Exercises

Squats

Squats are the most powerful single movement that can create a lower muscle and body power. Some tips to make your squats the most effective include deep squats (hips should be 90 degrees) and wide squats. Using as heavyweights as you can when you complete 4-10 reps for 2-3 sets.

Deadlifts

This is another excellent exercise that strengthens the hamstrings and glutes effectively. Again, lifting heavy is necessary to achieve the best results. When you rise, you can pinch your glutes and feel the burning as you hit the top.

Deadbug

Take a tabletop position with your arms raised directly above your head. Pull your ribs back, stretch. Then straighten down one leg while you lower the opposite arm: return and repeat. Try to complete 10-15 reps per set for 3-4 sets.

Hip Thrusts

The hip thrust is a must for anyone who wants to grow their booty. The resistance band around your knees can be used to stimulate your side glutes more. Support your upper back on a sofa, bed, or bench and place the lower part of your shoulder blades on the bench. Pull your feet in order to bring them under your knees. Keep your knees bent and move your hips to rise off the ground. You can adjust your feet to find the place where your glutes really activate the most. To increase the difficulty you can perform the exercise using a single leg at a time.

Donkey Kicks

A donkey kick is a typical glute-targeted move. You can attach a band to make the exercise more challenging. Get on all fours. Lift one foot up to the ceiling and bend your knee. Do not arch your back to raise your leg – continual hip/glute movement is key in this exercise. You need to activate your glute to lift your leg until your quad forms a symmetrical extension of your torso. Do not lift the thigh higher than the torso. Repeat for reps and switch to the other leg.

Floor Jacks

This variant of a jumping jack is likely to throw the glutes. Lay flat on the floor on your back or stomach. Arms and legs stretched out. Make sure your knees remain straight during movement, your feet and arms are off the floor and concentrate on relaxing the glutes. Extend the arms and legs to form an 'X' shape then return to the start position. Perform either 30-60 reps or complete as many as possible in 30-60 seconds for 3 sets.

The Uni-Leg Chair Squat

You start by sitting near a chair with crossed arms, chest raised, right foot firmly on the floor, and left leg raised by 8 inches. Engage your abs and slightly lean your body into standing. Push your right foot down into the floor, push your glutes backward (like in a normal squat), and straighten your knee right away, while pulling on your glutes, not to the full degree. Hold your left leg off the floor and balance for a three second count. Lower and repeat gradually. Do 2-4 sets of 10 reps on each leg.

Straight Leg Dumbbell Deadlift

Hold your dumbbells, arms by your side, feet hip-wide apart, legs straight. Hinge at the hips to lower your hands and upper body to the floor without bending your knees or rounding your back. Stop when you feel your glutes and hamstrings tight, then go back to the starting position.

Lunge Knee Raise

Stand upright with your feet shoulder width apart. Place your right leg back into the reverse lunge position, go as low as you can, keep your back straight and ensure that your knee doesn't hit the floor. Hold this lunge position for a three second count and push forward and up with your right leg until it is at a 90° from your torso.

Quadruped Hip Extension

Start on your hands and knees under your hips. Keeping the core muscles activated, raise the left leg gradually. When you bring your foot up to the ceiling, your knee will remain bent. Avoid moving or arching your back, keeping your core braced, and not moving your hips during the exercise. Straighten the lifted leg then return it to the lifted bent knee position and the to the floor to return to the start position, that's one rep. Repeat for the same leg for 8-12 reps and then change sides.

Booty Builder Workout Plan

You can create your own plan by following these steps:

- Choose 4-6 exercises
- Do as many exercises as you need to really feel the glutes working.
- Many exercises, like the single leg hip thrust, will only take 4-6 reps, while others, such as the squat, will allow you to do 10-12 repetitions for 3-5 sets.
- At least three days a week, perform a booty exercise.

Seven day booty builder plan

Day 1

Squats: 3 sets of 8-12 reps

Hip Thrust: 3 sets of 4-8 reps

Floor Jacks: 2 sets of 5-6 reps

Day 2

Deadlift: 3 sets of 4-6 reps

Donkey Kicks: 3 sets of 5-6 reps

Uni Leg Chair Squat: 3 sets of 4-6 reps

Day 3

Squats: 3 sets of 8–10 reps

Hip Thrusts: 2 set of 8–10 reps

Deadbug: 2 sets of 5-6 reps

Day 4

Quadruped Hip Extension: 3 sets of 8–10 reps

Donkey Kicks: 3 sets of 5-6 reps

Floor Jacks: 2 sets of 5-6 reps

Day 5

Squats: 3 sets of 8–10 reps

Lunge Knee Raise : 3 sets of 8–10 reps

Deadlift: 3 sets of 4-6 reps

Day 6

Hip Thrust: 3 sets of 8-10 reps

Uni leg chair squat: 3 sets of 4-6 reps

Deadbug: 2 sets of 5-6 reps

Day 7

Quadruped Hip extension: 3 sets of 8–10 reps

Straight Leg Dumbbell Deadlift: 2 sets of 5-6 reps

Donkey Kicks: 3 sets of 5-6 reps

Conclusion

Keep in mind that it might take a while and effort, but if all exercises performed correctly, it will all be worth it. A good flattening of the stomach is a matter of burning fat and muscle building. Cardiovascular workouts like running, walking, elliptical training, and cycling are the perfect way to lose body fat and to tone the legs. These exercises help you to burn the fat of your stomach, tone your legs, and build your booty.

All the exercises mentioned in this eBook provide you with a strong foundation for the weightless shaping of your body. Stay calm and feel the glutes burning after every exercise. Be sure that you have dumbbells, a resistance band, kettlebells, or similar equipment. Muscle building is focused on incremental overload, it is exhausting! If you want to optimize your success rate, before and after your exercise, you want to supplement with some protein and carbohydrates.

You can keep things easy with some fruit and protein shake for your pre-workout meal. You need to make sure that you eat a snack or a meal, depending on your lifestyle after training.